START FROM JOY GUIDED JOURNEY

START FROM
JOY

GUIDED JOURNEY

A Road Map to Emotional Health & Positive Change

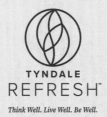

TYNDALE
REFRESH™

Think Well. Live Well. Be Well.

Visit Tyndale online at tyndale.com.

Visit the authors online at https://enjoycowellness.com.

Tyndale and Tyndale's quill logo are registered trademarks of Tyndale House Ministries. *Tyndale Refresh* and the Tyndale Refresh logo are trademarks of Tyndale House Ministries. Tyndale Refresh is a nonfiction imprint of Tyndale House Publishers, Carol Stream, Illinois.

Start from Joy Guided Journey

Edited by Stephanie Rische

Published in association with the literary agency of Legacy, LLC, 501 N. Orlando Avenue, Suite #313-348, Winter Park, FL 32789.

For information about special discounts for bulk purchases, please contact Tyndale House Publishers at csresponse@tyndale.com, or call 1-855-277-9400.

To protect the privacy of our clients, the names and details of our case examples have been changed. All names are fictional, and any resemblance between the composites and real people is coincidental.

Library of Congress Cataloging-in-Publication Data

A catalog record for this book is available from the Library of Congress.

ISBN 978-1-4964-6669-3

Printed in the United States of America

28	27	26	25	24	23	22
7	6	5	4	3	2	1

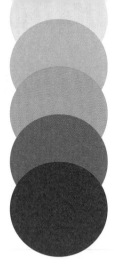

CONTENTS

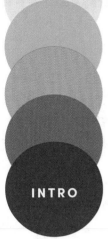

MAKING YOUR DREAM A REALITY

"START FROM JOY" IS AN APPROACH that has transformed our lives—and the lives of countless clients—for the better. It's not about choosing happiness, being blindly optimistic, having a positive mindset, or any other hokey misconceptions surrounding joy. Instead, it's the way to make positive changes—and to make them last.

We run an emotional health and wellness company called Enjoyco, where we see clients who want good things for their lives. They want to get a job that honors their passions. They want their bodies to be fit and healthy. They want their spiritual lives to be marked by fervor and enthusiasm. They want relationships that feed their soul. The problem is, they often start their quest for change with disempowering emotions like shame, guilt, and fear.

They're afraid of what will happen if they don't find a job soon. They shame themselves into going to the gym. They feel guilty if they miss a day of Bible reading. And these feelings of shame, guilt, and fear get in the way of intimacy in their relationships. These disempowering emotions sabotage them, creating patterns that lead them further from the change they want.

Starting from joy simply means putting empowering emotions—namely, joy—at the onset of positive change. Rather than believing joy will come after you change, you can embody joy at the *start* of change.

You might be thinking, *I don't struggle with shame, guilt, and fear.* But if you're stuck in old patterns, it's likely that disempowering emotions are under the surface. Maybe you want to change your relationship with your finances, but you keep spending blindly without creating a plan. You want to change the way you show up in your marriage and parenting, but you keep tuning out emotionally when your spouse or kids bring up hard topics. You want to have good boundaries at work, but any time your job gets stressful, you compromise and overwork. You've tried to change before, but no matter what you do, you keep getting stuck.

Not only that, but any results you've managed to accomplish are quick to disappear. The weight you lost from that last diet has all come back. The steps you took to decrease your dependence on your phone are now out the window. The habits you built to read your Bible and pray more have washed away in the busyness of life. You just haven't found a way to make positive change stick for you.

If this sounds like your story, we invite you to start from joy instead.

Over the years, we've studied how shame, guilt, and fear sabotage the change we want in life. We might experience shame for continually repeating harmful actions or for feeling certain emotions we think we shouldn't have. We might feel guilty for not being grateful enough for what we have. We might hear the voice of fear paralyzing us from taking the next right step. The way to counteract these emotions is to know the path back to joy.

Rather than believing joy will come after you change, you can embody joy at the *start* of change.

This is where the seven principles for starting from joy come in. They're meant to combat these disempowering emotions at every entry point so you can get back to joy in your journey to positive change. They are:

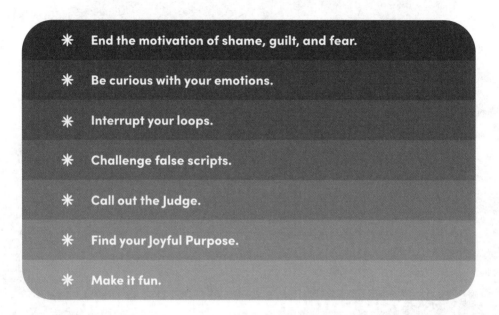

* **End the motivation of shame, guilt, and fear.**

* **Be curious with your emotions.**

* **Interrupt your loops.**

* **Challenge false scripts.**

* **Call out the Judge.**

* **Find your Joyful Purpose.**

* **Make it fun.**

We wrote the book *Start from Joy* to show anyone who's burned out from positive change that there can be a different approach. Instead of feeling pressure to change, you can embrace a lighter spirit. Instead of repeating old patterns, you can get rid of shame, guilt, and fear, and find lasting change. Instead of putting off joy to the future, you can build a fulfilling life today, before anything about your life changes.

The purpose of this guided journey is to help you put these principles into practice. We don't just want you to be inspired by these ideas; we want you to be able to apply them to your own life. In this book you'll find practical tools to help you experience the change you desire. We've developed these proprietary tools in our work at Enjoyco, and they have been successfully used by our clients. In this guided journey, you'll learn how to use tools such as the Negativity Loop, the Boundaries Planner, the W.I.L.L., and more.

HOW TO USE THIS BOOK

This guided journey is intended to be used in conjunction with the primary book, *Start from Joy*. We recommend reading *Start from Joy* first and then using the guided journey to apply the principles to your life in an area where you're seeking positive change, as it's helpful to know how all the principles work together when going through the guided journey. Or you can work through a session in this guidebook after reading the corresponding chapter in the main book. This is especially helpful if you're going through this guidebook with a group.

Each of the seven sessions focuses on a start-from-joy principle. Following a brief introduction to each principle, you'll find group discussion questions and an exercise to apply the principle to your circumstances.

This book can be used with a group or individually. After years of study, we've learned that joy is most often found in community. When we walk through life with others, joy becomes more real and tangible. We believe that when groups gather around these principles, they can make positive changes together.

That said, the guided journey can also be used on your own. If you're going through these sessions individually, we recommend carving out a quiet part of your day to do this work. Treat yourself to a coffee, find one of your favorite spots, and work through the group discussion questions as journal prompts. Then go through the exercises.

ARE YOU READY FOR A FRESH START?

A therapist friend once told me (Neal) that when you're sledding and you've been down a hill multiple times, your sled is almost forced to go down the path that's been carved in the snow. Committing to the work of healing, she said, is like pouring fresh snow on the hill so you're free to travel wherever you want to go.

That's our hope for you as you read *Start from Joy* and work through this guided journey: that this experience will be like pouring a fresh coat of snow on paths you've traveled for ages. You don't have to repeat old patterns. The past doesn't have to dictate your future. You can be free to travel wherever you want to go.

You can lay down the heavy burden you've been carrying so you can live lighter and freer . . . while also making your dreams a reality.

END THE MOTIVATION OF SHAME, GUILT, AND FEAR

A deeper look at chapters 1–2 of Start from Joy

CLAUDIA WAS HAVING A DAY.

It had started off well. She made it to work on time, with her favorite latte in hand. Her email wasn't overflowing, and her coworkers' spirits were light. But all it took was one meeting to derail her day. Her boss called out a mistake she'd made on a client project. Not only was this publicly humiliating, but she couldn't believe she'd done it in the first place.

Taking in her coworkers' judgmental glances, she told herself, *I'm so stupid. I have to do better.*

When Claudia got home, her day got worse. Already filled to the brim with negativity, she snapped at her two boys when they made a mess in the living room. They retreated to their rooms, feeling crushed. In her head, a familiar voice resounded, *I can't believe I did that. I have to do better.*

Now she felt flooded. An attempt to talk with her husband turned into a sharp dispute. He walked off, leaving her alone with her thoughts. *I'm scared we're growing apart. I have to do better.*

At work and at home, she wanted to do better, to *be* better. She wanted to have a strong relationship with her husband and her boys, and she wanted to feel confident at her job. But instead of offering herself the forgiveness and kindness that would make this change possible, she beat herself up. Like most of my (Carly's) clients, Claudia falsely believed that if she wasn't hard on herself for her mistakes, she wouldn't change.

What she didn't realize was that by using shame, guilt, and fear as motivators, she was only making positive change harder for herself.

A NEW APPROACH TO CHANGE

When I (Carly) introduce the start-from-joy approach to my clients, I teach them a new way to go about positive change. I help them remove the emotional charge of shame, guilt, and fear so they can pursue positive change with joy.

The concept might sound simple, but it doesn't happen automatically. Many of us don't want to—or don't know how to—let go of shame, guilt, and fear. We've spent too long in a self-improvement culture that preaches results above everything. We believe that if we let go of these negative emotions, we'll be "too soft" on ourselves and change won't happen. What we miss is that while pain is part of change, pain isn't a lasting motivator.

> When shame, guilt, and fear are motivators for change, they lead to self-sabotage.

We often use shame, guilt, and fear as motivators when we're looking for fast results. When the end result is all we care about, we're willing to employ any means to get it. To a degree, this strategy works. Yet inevitably it backfires. While shame, guilt, and fear can bring quick results, they don't lead to lasting, satisfying change—the kind you feel good about in the end.

For instance, someone might shame their body so they'll work out (*Ugh, I'm so fat. I need to go to the gym*). They might go to the gym but at the cost of wounding their view of themselves. Someone might guilt themselves into reading their Bible and praying because they forgot the day before (*I feel bad for missing my devotion time yesterday—I'll do better tomorrow*). They might check the box but at the cost of true intimacy with God. Or someone might scare themselves into anxiously pursuing their partner after feeling disconnected (*If I don't reach out to her, I'll lose her forever*). This might make them feel better in the moment but at the cost of denying the relationship the space it needs to grow.

When shame, guilt, and fear are motivators for change, they lead to self-sabotage.

TOXIC EMOTIONS VS. HEALTHY EMOTIONS

At this point, you may be wondering if these emotions of shame, guilt, and fear are all bad. The Bible says there's a positive side to these feelings when viewed through the right lens.

Shame can lead to repentance and humility. The healthy side of shame says we aren't enough on our own and points us in humility to Jesus. This truth is illustrated in Psalm 51:1-2: "Have mercy on me, O God, according to your unfailing love; according to your great compassion blot out my transgressions. Wash away all my iniquity and cleanse me from my sin."

Guilt can lead to forgiveness of sins. The healthy side of guilt acknowledges we've done wrong but points us to the grace of Jesus. The Bible says, "If we confess our sins to him, he is faithful and just to forgive us our sins and to cleanse us from all wickedness" (1 John 1:9, NLT).

Fear can lead to wisdom. The healthy side of fear says we can't fully plan our own way, but God is in control of everything. This is illustrated in Proverbs 9:10: "The fear of the LORD is the beginning of wisdom, and knowledge of the Holy One is understanding."

Yet most of the time, we don't use these emotions in the way the Bible points to. Instead . . .

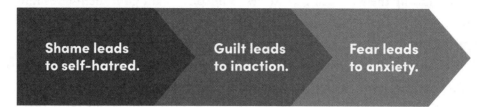

Shame leads to self-hatred.

Guilt leads to inaction.

Fear leads to anxiety.

Why do we hold on to the toxic side of these emotions? If Jesus washed away the shame that leads to self-hatred, why do we choose to remain in it? If he has cleansed our guilt, why do we continue to heap it on ourselves? And if his perfect love casts out fear, why do we let fear rule our lives?

We might hold on to shame, guilt, and fear because of what was modeled to us, because these emotions give us quick results, or because we bond with others over them. We assume that holding on to these emotions in our positive-change journey will put us in control of our lives. But shame, guilt, and fear are healthy only when they lead us back to God. Toxic shame, guilt, and fear, on the other hand, point us back to ourselves. When we motivate ourselves with these emotions, we buy into the idea that we have complete power to change ourselves.

> Shame, guilt, and fear are healthy only when they lead us back to God.

The more we try to be the saviors of our own life, the more we pile on the pressure to change. It's to this end that Jesus says, "Come to me, all of you who are weary and carry heavy burdens, and I will give you rest. Take my yoke upon you. Let me teach you, because I am humble and gentle at heart, and you will find rest for your souls. For my yoke is easy to bear, and the burden I give you is light."[1]

Jesus' heart is to take the burden of toxic shame, guilt, and fear away from us. The first principle for starting from joy is to end these motivations entirely so we can live fully in the freedom Christ gives us. It's from this place of freedom that we achieve lasting positive change.

 GROUP DISCUSSION QUESTIONS

1. In *Start from Joy*, we offer definitions for shame, guilt, fear, and joy (see the introduction). How would you define these emotions in your own words?

2. Do you fear that if you go easy on yourself, you won't change? Where do you think this idea comes from?

3. How do you balance your personal agency (your responsibility to act) with trust in God?

4. Can you share about a time when you experienced change that stuck? What do you attribute that positive change to?

5. Think about Jesus' promise that his yoke is easy and his burden is light (Matthew 11:28-30, NLT). What would it look like for you to pursue change with this perspective in mind?

6. Have you been part of groups in the past that have used shame, guilt, and fear as motivators for change? What were the results, both long-term and short-term?

EXERCISE: EXPLORE YOUR MOTIVATIONS

You can answer the following questions using the blank spaces provided to determine how shame, guilt, and fear have guided your journey toward positive change to this point and what you need to move forward. Answer these questions individually.

LOOKING BACK

Claudia's reliance on old motivators could only change once she got clarity on how they hadn't worked in the past. Reflect on how these motivators have showed up in your positive-change journeys.

When was a time you felt pressured to change?

What did you do to try to bring about this change?

What emotions drove this desire to change?

What setbacks did you experience during this process?
How did you respond to those challenges?

Did you achieve results? If so, how long did the change last?

What patterns do you notice about your quest for positive change?

LOOKING FORWARD

Claudia didn't want to be hard on herself—she simply didn't know any other way. When she worked with me (Carly), we got to the root of the emotions driving her self-sabotage. Eventually she was able to recognize these patterns in her life, and she realized that being hard on herself wasn't working. Instead of looking back, she started envisioning the future she hoped for. How did she want to approach these circumstances in the future? What would it look like if she weren't hard on herself and instead quickly returned to joy?

You, too, can shift your thinking to your desires for the future. When you clarify what you want and how you want to feel, the destination becomes clearer.

What is something you currently want to change in your life?
Write out your specific goal.

Imagine that you did it. You achieved this positive change without beating yourself up or using shame, guilt, and fear as motivators. You centered yourself around joy and changed your life in a way that felt great all the way through. You handled setbacks with joy. Now write a congratulations letter to your future self, detailing the steps you took and the way it felt to reach this milestone.

Let's make

the past a memory

and the future

a reality.

BE CURIOUS WITH YOUR EMOTIONS

A deeper look at chapter 3 of Start from Joy

WHEN I (NEAL) WAS IN SEMINARY, I wanted to explore my dream of writing a novel. So in that first year, when I was settling into deep theological studies and a new season of life, I did just that—I wrote a book. And then I somehow convinced the seminary to let me work one-on-one with a professor to edit my book for a course credit. I thought it would be the easiest course of my seminary career . . . that is, until I turned in my manuscript.

Dr. Adams was well-versed in literature and its intersection with theology. Before we started working on my manuscript together, we had long conversations about C. S. Lewis and his life as a writer. She knew everything about him, from his writing routines to the influences behind his books. If anyone was going to help me refine this manuscript, it was her.

After she read the manuscript, she tore it apart—in the gentlest way, of course.

"I love your ideas," she started off.

"But?" I knew it was coming.

"But . . . your main character is flat."

"What do you mean?"

"I mean he doesn't experience anything. He has no emotions about things that should bother him."

I read through the manuscript that night and realized she was right. I had accidentally written my main character to have no real emotions. His demeanor was calm throughout the arc of the story, letting the action of the narrative pull him forward rather than experiencing any sort of character development.

Here's the thing: the main character was based on me. *I* wasn't allowing myself to feel strong emotions.

As I worked with my professor, I came to realize that the best stories have characters that move, feel, and change. My character seemed to be above it all—like he wasn't part of the real world.

I used to think people needed to be mentally tough, stoic, and emotionally rigid (like the character in my novel) to experience lasting change. But Jesus didn't fit that picture—he wasn't above it all. Jesus became fully human,[1] which means he had emotions, just like we do.

I have come to understand since then that emotions don't hold us back; they propel us to our greatest changes in life. The solution isn't to build dams around our emotions, causing them to flood when those protections falter, but to let them flow freely and safely.

NAMING AND VALIDATING EMOTIONS

If you numb one emotion, you numb them all.

One thing I (Carly) often tell my clients is that if you numb one emotion, you numb them all. You can't numb anger and then expect to experience the fullness of joy. You can't bury "negative" emotions and only embrace positive ones. In *Start from Joy*, we talk in depth about the tyranny of toxic positivity (see chapter 3). If you don't feel safe exploring all your emotions, you can never experience true joy.

In the Bible, Jesus doesn't back away from the full breadth of his emotions. He felt both anger and grief over the death of his friend Lazarus, even though he knew he'd raise Lazarus from the dead.[2] Jesus expressed his righteous anger by overturning tables in the Temple courts.[3] He felt deep sorrow in the garden of Gethsemane, knowing the suffering that lay ahead.[4] Jesus didn't steer away from hard emotions, yet he experienced the fullness of joy.[5]

> Allowing ourselves to feel all our emotions leads to deeper joy.

Allowing ourselves to feel all our emotions leads to deeper joy. A start-from-joy approach is not toxic positivity; it's not pasting a happy smile on everything. Rather, it's learning from the breadth of our feelings.

Being curious with our emotions means giving them space so we can learn from them—*all* of them. When we don't acknowledge our emotions, we end up reacting to them in unhealthy ways and self-sabotaging. If you want to bring empowering emotions into your journey toward change, you have to get curious about all your emotions instead of trying to select only the ones you want to keep.

In chapter 3 of *Start from Joy*, we talk about being curious with your emotions. This entails naming them, regulating them, learning from them, and validating them. This can be a challenging process, especially if you've been told that your emotions are too much or too dramatic, or that they aren't real. Maybe you've spent a lifetime hiding your emotions. If that's you, it's possible to learn to embrace all your emotions and feel safe with them.

GROUP DISCUSSION QUESTIONS

1. Consider passages such as Matthew 21:12, John 11:1-44, and John 17:13. What do you notice about the way Jesus deals with emotions? How does this compare with the way you were taught to handle emotions?

2. Describe your relationship with emotions. Do you feel free to embrace all your emotions, or are there some you'd rather not feel? What emotions do you struggle with?

3. Recall a time someone discounted your feelings by minimizing them, invalidating them, ignoring them, expressing toxic positivity, or telling you not to feel a certain way. How did it affect your situation? How did it feel to have your emotions dismissed?

4. Recall a time someone held space for your feelings by validating them, affirming them, listening nonjudgmentally, showing empathy, or saying, "That's really difficult—tell me more." How did it affect your situation? How did it feel to have your emotions accepted?

5. Do you have to agree with or completely understand someone's feelings to respect and validate them? Why or why not? Why do you think it's difficult to do this?

6. Think about the way emotions were treated in your family when you were growing up. What do you appreciate about it? What would you want to change?

7. Think about a recent time you felt a strong emotion. What does that emotion say about what you value?

EXERCISE: EMOTIONAL SAFETY ASSESSMENT

Create a list of people, places, and practices that help you feel safe with your emotions.

PEOPLE
Who are the safe people in your life—
the ones you can trust with your emotions?

PLACES

What places do you like to go to (in your mind or physically) that help you feel grounded, safe, and secure?

PRACTICES

What practices help you self-regulate when your emotions feel overwhelming (for example, deep breathing, prayer, etc.)?

When

emotions are fully felt,

realized, and processed,

they can help us reclaim

our sense of

agency.

INTERRUPT YOUR LOOPS

A deeper look at chapter 4 of Start from Joy

AT 9 P.M. EASTERN TIME ON MARCH 7, 1965, around 48 million Americans were glued to their television sets. Airing on ABC was the television premiere of *Judgment at Nuremberg*, a star-studded film about the trials of Nazi judges who paved the way for the oppression of Jews. The huge viewing audience was appalled that humans could be complicit in such evil.

Minutes after the movie started, it was interrupted by a breaking news broadcast. What Americans saw next horrified them.[1]

More than six hundred civil rights activists marched across the Edmund Pettus Bridge in Selma, Alabama, led by a young John Lewis. As they reached the crest of the bridge, they were met by a blockade of state troopers. The mayor ordered them to stop, but they marched on, resolute.

Moments later, the troopers charged. Tear gas and screams pierced the air. Americans in the audience were horrified by the evil in their own country. Cameras that captured the event showed troopers beating marchers who weren't fighting back. The people who were watching didn't want to be like the Nazi judges who allowed evil to prevail. They wanted change to happen.[2]

"Bloody Sunday," as the day came to be called, was the greatest test of the nonviolent response for the civil rights movement. The public outrage that stemmed from the broadcast paved the way for the Voting Rights Act to be passed later that year. Richard Cohen, an attorney with the Southern Poverty Law Center, said, "The violence was being perpetrated by the oppressors, not the oppressed, and that was an incredibly powerful message and an incredibly important tool during the movement."[3]

Through the teachings of Martin Luther King Jr., the activists understood that if they gave in to the natural temptation to fight back after being struck, they would sabotage their cause. They had to interrupt the pattern. In doing so, they paved the way for positive change.

GETTING UNSTUCK FROM YOUR PATTERNS

Interrupting patterns is holy work, and the power to break those natural temptations isn't found solely within ourselves. When we tap into supernatural joy, we're able to persevere, break past our default settings, and create lasting change.

Interrupting patterns is holy work.

We've all experienced emotional patterns that sabotage our ability to change. In *Start from Joy*, we talk about the Negativity Loop, a tool we developed to help clients understand their patterns (see chapter 4). First we experience a stressor, then a negative thought, then a hard emotion. To escape the hard emotion, we have a protection response. As we keep repeating our protection response, our patterns compound. Our stressors feel bigger, and we feel more shame, more fear, and more guilt-driven thoughts. These responses produce more overwhelming emotions, which require an even bigger protection response to overcome.

Maybe you struggle with a binge protection response of overworking when you feel anxious or fearful. Or maybe you default to an avoidance protection response when money worries come up. Or perhaps you have a rage protection response when your spouse triggers one of your insecurities. Lasting change is on the other side . . . if you can interrupt these loops.

Interrupting your patterns might seem impossible at first. But let me encourage you: you're not doing this work alone. The Holy Spirit inside you is empowering you for change. In the following group discussion questions and exercise, you'll gain awareness of your Negativity Loop so you can begin the holy work of breaking these patterns.

 GROUP DISCUSSION QUESTIONS

1. Do you know of someone who has successfully broken their unhealthy patterns? If so, how did they do it?

2. How comfortable are you with getting feedback about your patterns? What circumstances make it easier to receive feedback?

3. When you feel anxious, guilt-ridden, angry, or ashamed, what do you reach for to soothe the pain? When you feel restless, empty, lonely, or lost, what do you do to try to fill the emptiness? What are you trying to find protection from?

4. What's a wise action you can take to interrupt your loops?
   (Remember, binge responses need boundaries, avoidance
   responses need attention, and rage responses need reconnection.)

5. What new life do you think is waiting for you on the other side of
   breaking your loop?

6. Think about a pattern you've been trying to interrupt for a long time. What results would indicate that you're truly interrupting the pattern and not just muscling your way into temporary change? Check out Galatians 5:22-23 for a list of the fruit of the Spirit. When you see this kind of fruit in your life, you'll know you're on the right track!

EXERCISE: CREATE YOUR NEGATIVITY LOOP

The Negativity Loop is a tool that helps you gain clarity over the emotional patterns that are sabotaging your quest for positive change. This exercise will guide you through the process of creating a Negativity Loop.

First, think about an area of your life where you want to experience dramatic transformation. This could be in the area of health, relationships, faith, work, finances, or something else.

Maybe you feel disconnected from your spouse and you want to enjoy your marriage again. Or maybe you feel disappointed with your health and you want to enjoy feeding your body with proper nutrition. Maybe debt has taken a toll on you and you want to experience a breakthrough in your financial situation.

Write down the specific change you'd like to see in your life.

List all the stressors that produce subsequent stress in this area of your life.
Here are some examples:

- comparison with thin people around you
- your mom's comments about your singleness during the holidays
- not knowing how to handle a new project at work
- your child getting in trouble at school
- missing your devotion time for the day

Once you've made a list of stressors, choose one to create a Negativity Loop around (see the Negativity Loop at the end of this session). Write it down in the stressor portion of the loop. Then, in the thoughts portion, write how you would respond to the stressor. Here are some examples of thoughts that might follow a stressor:

- *If only I had a body like hers.*
- *Another reminder that I'm still alone. Why hasn't anyone chosen me?*
- *I'm not capable of completing this project. Everyone will judge me.*
- *I'm a failure as a parent. I'm losing my child.*
- *I'm a terrible Christian. Why would God love me?*

Behind each of these thoughts is a false script—a misleading idea about what brings us joy. In the thoughts portion of your Negativity Loop, underneath your response to the stressor, write down the false script that powers your critical thoughts. Here are some examples of false scripts:

- *I'll be happy after I lose the weight.*
- *If I were married, then I'd be happy.*

- *I would be happy if I didn't have to do hard work.*
- *I need perfect relationships with my kids to be happy.*
- *If I were a better Christian, then I'd be happy.*

What emotion do you experience as a result of your negative thoughts? It could be shame, guilt, fear, anxiety, overwhelm, sadness, anger, or something else. In the emotions portion of your loop, write down the emotion. Try to be as specific as possible when labeling this feeling.

Finally, write down the protection you seek to feel better. Common protections include bingeing, avoidance, and rage responses. Binge protections include overworking, overeating, overexercising, overreacting, and overthinking. Avoidance protections include disengaging, procrastinating, watching Netflix, and ignoring what you need to do. Rage protections include complaining, blaming someone else, and exploding on social media. Write this down in the protection portion of your Negativity Loop.

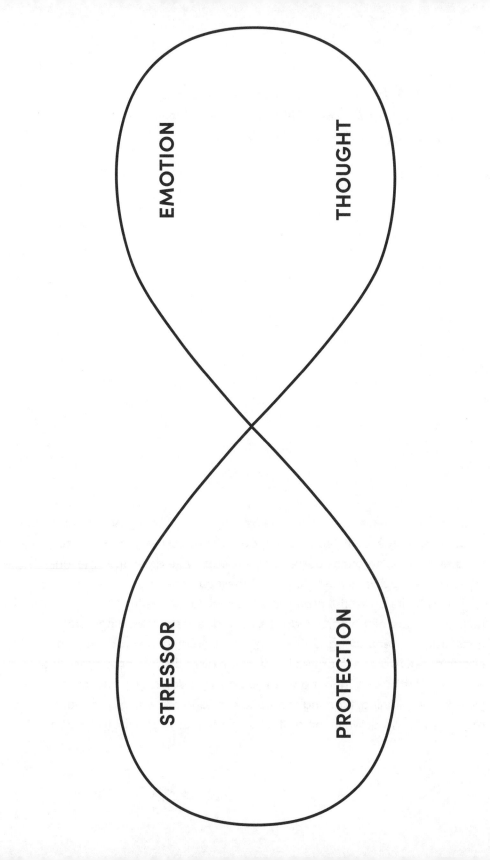

Patterns you are blind to

are patterns you repeat.

SESSION 4

CHALLENGE FALSE SCRIPTS

A deeper look at chapter 5 of Start from Joy

WHEN NEAL AND I WERE ENGAGED and both attending seminary, he called me and asked if I would swing by his apartment so he could tell me something. When I walked in wearing a slightly concerned smile, I found him pacing the room, as if he were rehearsing a speech. He sat me down and delivered the news.

He was quitting seminary.

Not only that, but he was going to become an entrepreneur.

Oh, and our wedding was in *one month*. The perfect time to uproot his entire life.

I wasn't a fan of the idea at first. We went back and forth, debating whether a master's degree would help him in his career. We tried to discern where God was leading him and what this would mean for our newlywed life. After much discussion, we felt strongly that God was lighting up a passion in Neal's heart. What wasn't clear to me, however, was the timing.

I could see his motivation for doing this just one month before the wedding. Now that we were about to get married, he'd convinced himself he had to be a provider. He felt he had to measure up to a script in his head—that having a happy marriage meant making lots of money.

Neal ended up leaving seminary to follow God's calling for him in the world of business. But the script in his head—the one that had him constantly trying to hustle, strive, and measure up—got in the way of this calling and caused him to burn out.

Neal bought into what we call a false script—believing you'll find happiness and joy from a source that will never be able to deliver. False scripts twist and distort our beautiful desires. They make happiness conditional on something apart from God. We try to find joy through losing weight, getting out of debt, finding a partner, or checking off the box of being a good Christian. Our families, our friends, our culture, and our traumatic experiences convince us that if we measure up to the call to do better and be better, then we'll have joy.

But God wants us to experience joy *now*, before we change anything about our lives. God wants our joy to grow like a tidal wave, sweeping others into it as well.

Jesus never said anything about life becoming meaningful once we lose weight. He didn't say we'll have joy once we get disciplined about our finances. He didn't say we need to find a spouse to experience a fulfilling life. Jesus compelled us to put our hope in only one thing: we are to seek his Kingdom, not what others worry about. Then everything else we need will come to us.[1]

But God wants us to experience joy *now*.

When we put our hope in the wrong things, it's no wonder we feel disappointed, burned out, and fearful. The things we're pursuing were never meant to be our hope; they were never meant to give us joy.

Joy is not a destination but a posture. Once we assume this posture, our greatest change will open up to us. We'll enjoy increased health and improved relationships. Our finances will no longer weigh on us like a ball and chain. We'll engage with our jobs at a deeper level and find more satisfaction in our work.

> **Joy is not a destination but a posture.**

In the grand scheme of things, our positive-change journey is less about ourselves and more about what God wants to do through us. When we tie ourselves to the larger purpose of what God is doing, we will realize that joy is possible today, even if we don't change.

You don't need to work harder, try harder, or burden yourself to experience joy.

You don't need to hustle to change the unworthy parts of yourself.

And you don't need to put your hope in changing your status when it comes to weight, money, or relationships. Instead, you can invest in a bigger hope that puts everything else into perspective.

When we plug into a bigger story, we can step back and see everything in its proper place. In other words, we don't have to try so hard.

To reclaim the joy in positive change, we have to battle our false scripts. The following group discussion questions and exercise will help you uncover your false scripts and create boundaries to protect yourself from their influence.

? GROUP DISCUSSION QUESTIONS

1. Recall the advertisements you've noticed recently on social media, TV, or the radio. Take a few moments to analyze one.

   A. *What is the ad selling? What problem is it trying to solve?*

   B. *Where does the ad suggest you can find joy, happiness, or fulfillment? How is the product supposed to help you achieve that?*

C. *If you made this purchase, would you experience joy? If so, for how long?*

D. *Who profits when you make this purchase?*

2. Think through the main plot points of a "happily ever after" movie, TV show, or book. What life script does it suggest for achieving a happy ending?

3. If you feel comfortable sharing with the group, is there a false script you tend to buy into? What is it? How do you know it's a false script?

4. Identify something you long for that is a good desire. How can you tell whether your relationship with that desire is appropriate or idolatrous?

5. What's one small step you can take to reconnect to your values and decide what really matters to you?

6. What is one strategy from the boundaries section in chapter 5 of *Start from Joy* that stood out to you? How can you use this strategy when a false script triggers your shame, guilt, or fear?

7. How do you think your life would change if you were able to successfully identify a false script and then set a boundary to protect yourself?

EXERCISE: IDENTIFY FALSE SCRIPTS

Using the following exercise, identify your false scripts in the area you desire change.

POSITIVE-CHANGE AREA
In what area of life do you desire positive change?

Health

FALSE SCRIPT #1
What false script have you bought into in this area of your life?

I have to avoid looking and feeling older if I want to be happy.

EMOTION
What emotions does this false script result in?

Fear

ORIGIN
Where did this false script come from?

☑ family
☐ social groups
☐ culture and media
☐ trauma
☐ other: _____

EXPLORE
Write about your earliest memory (or a recent memory) that relates to this false script. When did this false script feel real for you?

I remember watching my parents suffer from health problems as they got older, and I don't want the same for myself. I will do whatever it takes to avoid feeling and looking older.

SAMPLE

On the following pages, identify a few false scripts in your own life.

POSITIVE-CHANGE AREA
In what area of life do you desire positive change?

FALSE SCRIPT #1
What false script have you bought into in this area of your life?

EMOTION
What emotions does this false script result in?

ORIGIN
Where did this false script come from?

☐ family
☐ social groups
☐ culture and media
☐ trauma
☐ other: _____

EXPLORE
Write about your earliest memory (or a recent memory) that relates to this false script. When did this false script feel real for you?

POSITIVE-CHANGE AREA
In what area of life do you desire positive change?

FALSE SCRIPT #2
What false script have you bought into in this area of your life?

EMOTION
What emotions does this false script result in?

ORIGIN
Where did this false script come from?

☐ family
☐ social groups
☐ culture and media
☐ trauma
☐ other: _____

EXPLORE
Write about your earliest memory (or a recent memory) that relates to this false script. When did this false script feel real for you?

POSITIVE-CHANGE AREA
In what area of life do you desire positive change?

FALSE SCRIPT #3
What false script have you bought into in this area of your life?

EMOTION
What emotions does this false script result in?

ORIGIN
Where did this false script come from?

☐ family
☐ social groups
☐ culture and media
☐ trauma
☐ other: _____

EXPLORE
Write about your earliest memory (or a recent memory) that relates to this false script. When did this false script feel real for you?

POSITIVE-CHANGE AREA
In what area of life do you desire positive change?

FALSE SCRIPT #4
What false script have you bought into in this area of your life?

EMOTION
What emotions does this false script result in?

ORIGIN
Where did this false script come from?

- ☐ family
- ☐ social groups
- ☐ culture and media
- ☐ trauma
- ☐ other: _____

EXPLORE
Write about your earliest memory (or a recent memory) that relates to this false script. When did this false script feel real for you?

POSITIVE-CHANGE AREA
In what area of life do you desire positive change?

FALSE SCRIPT #5
What false script have you bought into in this area of your life?

EMOTION
What emotions does this false script result in?

ORIGIN
Where did this false script come from?

- ☐ family
- ☐ social groups
- ☐ culture and media
- ☐ trauma
- ☐ other: _____

EXPLORE
Write about your earliest memory (or a recent memory) that relates to this false script. When did this false script feel real for you?

EXERCISE: BOUNDARIES PLANNER

Now that you've identified these false scripts, let's create some boundaries to protect you from their influence.

- **Who/what triggers this false script?** It could be specific people, friend groups, or social media accounts.
- **What upsets you about these people/influences?** What actions or circumstances create stress for you? Be as specific as you can.
- **What value needs protecting?** Once you identify what upsets you, ask yourself, *Why?* What value is this person or thing brushing up against?
- **What boundary strategy can help you protect what you value?** Refer to the strategies in chapter 5 of *Start from Joy* to determine which strategy can help you protect yourself.

Using the following example, complete the boundaries planner for the false scripts you identified.

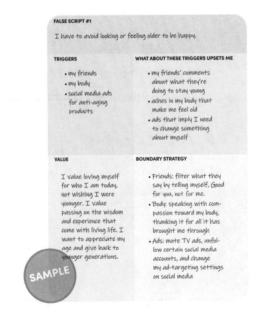

FALSE SCRIPT #1

I have to avoid looking or feeling older to be happy.

TRIGGERS

- my friends
- my body
- social media ads for anti-aging products

WHAT ABOUT THESE TRIGGERS UPSETS ME

- my friends' comments about what they're doing to stay young
- aches in my body that make me feel old
- ads that imply I need to change something about myself

VALUE

I value loving myself for who I am today, not wishing I were younger. I value passing on the wisdom and experience that come with living life. I want to appreciate my age and give back to younger generations.

BOUNDARY STRATEGY

- Friends: filter what they say by telling myself, Good for you, not for me.
- Body: speaking with compassion toward my body, thanking it for all it has brought me through
- Ads: mute TV ads, unfollow certain social media accounts, and change my ad-targeting settings on social media

SAMPLE

FALSE SCRIPT #1

TRIGGERS

WHAT ABOUT THESE TRIGGERS UPSETS ME

VALUE

BOUNDARY STRATEGY

FALSE SCRIPT #2

TRIGGERS

WHAT ABOUT THESE TRIGGERS UPSETS ME

VALUE

BOUNDARY STRATEGY

FALSE SCRIPT #3

TRIGGERS

WHAT ABOUT THESE TRIGGERS UPSETS ME

VALUE

BOUNDARY STRATEGY

FALSE SCRIPT #4

TRIGGERS

WHAT ABOUT THESE TRIGGERS UPSETS ME

VALUE

BOUNDARY STRATEGY

FALSE SCRIPT #5

TRIGGERS

WHAT ABOUT THESE TRIGGERS UPSETS ME

VALUE

BOUNDARY STRATEGY

The LORD is
my chosen
portion and my
cup; you hold my lot. The lines have
fallen for me in pleasant places;
indeed, I have a beautiful inheritance.

Psalm 16:5-6, ESV

CALL OUT THE JUDGE

A deeper look at chapter 6 of Start from Joy

"CARLY, I KNOW COGNITIVELY THAT GOD LOVES ME. But why don't I feel it?"

Tears flooded Young-Mi's eyes as she spoke. Something was making her feel stuck and unlovable before God. She knew that in order to get to the bottom of this she'd need to dig into her past, but she couldn't mine those territories on her own.

"When was a time you didn't feel loved?" I asked in our first session.

Her answer was almost instant. "With my family. I know my mom loved me, but I don't remember *feeling* her love for me."

Young-Mi's mom was dismissive and hard to please. She did everything a mother was expected to do—she fed and clothed her daughter, and she cleaned up around the house. She expected Young-Mi to get good grades and to do her chores. She often remarked on ways her daughter could improve, and only occasionally, when Young-Mi excelled at something, gave a small nod of her head and a "humph."

"As strange as it sounds, I craved that reaction," she told me. "It was the only time I knew I was okay in my mom's eyes."

As we spoke more about their relationship, it became clear why she didn't feel God's love.

"Is it possible that you imagine God to be like your mother?"

There were more tears. Then Young-Mi whispered, "Yes."

To Young-Mi, God's voice was judgmental and condemning, calling out her wrongdoing and only rarely giving her nods of approval. To her, God didn't feel warm, tenderhearted, and gentle; he seemed cold and distant.

This voice guided Young-Mi's life, telling her that she wasn't good enough, that she messed up a work assignment, that she had to measure up or she would face scorn. This voice was quick to label everything she did as bad or good, causing her shame, guilt, and fear to compound. She wanted good things for her life, but this voice—the one she assumed was God's voice—paralyzed her steps to positive change.

THE VOICE OF THE JUDGE

At Enjoyco, we see many clients who struggle with the voice of their inner critic. We call this voice "the Judge." The Judge tells us what we should and shouldn't do. It's intended to help us survive; the problem is that it's been overtaken by misguided expectations from our culture, our families, and our own stories. The Judge's voice has been tainted by our false scripts. As a result, the Judge labels the wrong things as good and bad. Here are some examples of the Judge's voice:

- *Having too much money is bad. Having a modest amount of money is good.*
- *Eating too many carbs is bad. Eating salads is good.*

- *Waiting to have kids is bad. Starting a family early is good.*
- *Sleeping in is bad. Reading your Bible every day is good.*
- *Struggling with anxiety is bad. Being happy is good.*

These judgments add a negative emotional charge to our positive-change journey. We feel shame if we get a raise. We feel guilty if we break our diet. We feel fear if our family doesn't look the way our parents expected. We feel like bad Christians if we don't open our Bible every day. And we feel like we're failing if we experience anxiety.

The reason these indictments paralyze us is because we live in a world full of gray. We don't have the luxury of choosing circumstances that are all good and avoiding circumstances that are all bad. Not all of these areas are moral issues—some are just a matter of preference. And fortunately, there's abundant grace from a loving God to cover any time we don't live up to what's good.

> To start from joy instead of shame, guilt, and fear, we have to call out this voice.

To start from joy instead of shame, guilt, and fear, we have to call out this voice. When we call out the Judge, we remove the emotional charge in our stressors. It's possible to view our stressors as neutral, not inherently bad. This neutrality levels out our emotional responses so we can stop shame, guilt, and fear, and break our old patterns.

Here's the freeing truth: the voice that's condemning you is not God. The Bible says, "There is now no condemnation for those who are in Christ Jesus."[1] Jesus came into the world not to condemn it, but to free it.[2] The Judge's voice urges you to measure up to your false scripts in the hope of experiencing joy someday, but God's voice gives you the freedom to experience joy *today*.

The following group discussion questions and exercise will help you find freedom from the clutches of the Judge.

GROUP DISCUSSION QUESTIONS

1. Do you relate to Young-Mi's version of God? In what ways is your Judge's voice similar and different?

2. How can you tell when the voice in your head is the voice of the Judge? What happens when you listen to that voice?

3. In chapter 6 of *Start from Joy*, we talk about how the Judge's voice has been overtaken by our culture, our families, and our own stories. If you feel comfortable sharing with the group, where did your Judge's voice come from?

4. The Judge's voice isn't all bad; it's just that it has been corrupted. What is the good part of that voice? In what ways does it protect you?

5. What false script is behind your Judge's voice?

6. How would the voice of Jesus counter your Judge's voice? Think of what Jesus might say about specific scenes from your life.

7. How can you call out the Judge's voice in your everyday life? How might you think and behave differently without the influence of this voice?

EXERCISE: THE JUDGE SCRIPT

To call out the Judge's voice, we need to know what it sounds like. In the following exercise, you can think through the false scripts you identified in session 4.

In what ways is the Judge critical of you?

What actions, qualities, or ideas does the Judge label as bad?

In the following chart, list the Judge's lies. Then note how the compassionate, gentle, and loving voice of Jesus would counteract this voice. Finally, write the truth that Jesus' voice reveals to you.

You can use this example to get started.

FALSE SCRIPT

I will be happy once I lose weight.

THE JUDGE SAYS . . .

- I should avoid carbs at all costs.
- Going to the gym is good.
- If I eat bad foods, I have to make up for it.
- I will be loved if I keep the weight off.

JESUS SAYS . . .

- Everything God created is good (1 Timothy 4:4).
- Godliness matters more than going to the gym (1 Timothy 4:8).
- There is no condemnation in Christ (Romans 8:1).
- Nothing can separate me from Christ's love (Romans 8:35).

THE TRUTH IS . . .

I can practice freedom and enjoyment in my eating and exercise, knowing that God loves me no matter what. What I eat doesn't make me good or bad in God's eyes. I am loved regardless of what I change about myself.

SAMPLE

FALSE SCRIPT

THE JUDGE SAYS . . .

JESUS SAYS . . .

THE TRUTH IS . . .

FALSE SCRIPT

THE JUDGE SAYS . . .

JESUS SAYS . . .

THE TRUTH IS . . .

FALSE SCRIPT

THE JUDGE SAYS . . .

JESUS SAYS . . .

THE TRUTH IS . . .

FALSE SCRIPT

THE JUDGE SAYS . . .

JESUS SAYS . . .

THE TRUTH IS . . .

FALSE SCRIPT

THE JUDGE SAYS . . .

JESUS SAYS . . .

THE TRUTH IS . . .

The next time

the Judge tries to call

you out on your mess,

call it out first. Say, "That's just

my Judge speaking," and then

move on. You have more

important things

to do.

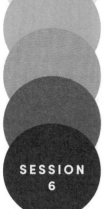

FIND YOUR JOYFUL PURPOSE

A deeper look at chapter 7 of Start from Joy

ON THE NIGHT BEFORE THEIR WEDDING, many grooms either party it up or pace around the room, worrying about the life change ahead. I (Neal) did neither of these things. In fact, I was surprisingly calm. I told my grooms-men and family I just wanted to do one thing: sit in my hotel room and finish reading *Man's Search for Meaning* by Viktor Frankl.

Reading about the Holocaust might sound like a morbid thing to do the night before my wedding, but I wanted my marriage to have a deeper mean-ing. I didn't want this new stage to be about my own happiness; I wanted it to serve a purpose beyond myself. I had seen my parents' marriage end because each person wanted something different for their own happiness. I wanted to break this pattern.

In his theory of logotherapy, Frankl presented the idea that life asks some-thing special of us; we do not ask anything of life. In other words, we make a life meaningful not by what we take from it but by what we give to it. This resonated with my desire to align with what God is doing in the world instead of pursuing a self-centered ambition. I'd seen too many couples make marriage about themselves and what they could get out of the relationship. We've been sold the false script that the point of marriage is to make us happy. I wanted something different for my marriage to Carly. I wanted us to serve a purpose that was bigger than ourselves.

When pain and trauma enter our stories, it's easy to forget our larger purpose. Our perspective shrinks, and we turn to false scripts that tell us we need to focus only on ourselves to be happy.

But pain doesn't have to make us self-focused. It's possible to take our pain and turn it outward. Instead of running from our wounds, we can turn them into a purpose that inspires and motivates us.

> We become what has our attention.

Someone once told me we become what has our attention. Before I got married, my attention gravitated toward the fear that I would mess up my marriage and get divorced like my parents had. But the more this fear captivated my attention, the more I brought fearful habits into my relationships. I needed a bigger purpose for my marriage.

FINDING YOUR JOYFUL PURPOSE

In chapter 7 of *Start from Joy*, we talk about a Joyful Purpose—the authentic reason behind our desire for positive change. Your Joyful Purpose fills you with passion. It relieves the burden to change and instead infuses your journey with joy.

In the Gospels we see that Jesus' entire life was fueled by purpose. His purpose clarified his steps. It slowed his pace. It highlighted his priorities. There was nothing reactive to what he did; everything was an intentional step toward fulfilling his mission. He lived on purpose.

In our journey to change, many of us live reactively. We desire change because we don't want to be like our parents or because we fear being overweight or because we hope to escape financial dependence. We're busy running from something negative instead of running toward something joyful.

Creating a Joyful Purpose is about articulating the motivation and vision for your life. In the following group discussion questions and exercise, you'll explore this bigger purpose so you can add joy into your journey to change.

 GROUP DISCUSSION QUESTIONS

1. Can you relate to Neal's story about wanting to break his parents' cycle when it came to his own marriage? Are there any cycles from your culture or family upbringing that you want to break?

2. In chapter 7 of *Start from Joy*, we talk about how having a Joyful Purpose helps cut through the comparison trap. When was the last time you compared yourself to someone else? How do you think having a Joyful Purpose would help in an instance like that?

3. Reflect on how Jesus lived out his purpose. We're called to live with intentionality too. Why do you think he was able to live so intentionally? What challenges tend to get in the way when we try to do the same?

4. Think about your life ten years from now. What do you want your life to look like? What are you doing now to become that person?

5. What are the benefits of having a Joyful Purpose? What are the fruits of such a purpose?

6. Think of a time you walked through something difficult. Did you have a larger purpose that helped you get through? If you feel comfortable, share this story with the group.

EXERCISE: A.I.M. FOR YOUR JOYFUL PURPOSE

Now it's time to define your Joyful Purpose.

A Joyful Purpose is the opposite of a false script. Sometimes we seek change because we want to fit cultural standards or meet family expectations. A Joyful Purpose is the authentic reason you want change—a reason that goes beyond what other people desire for your life. It's a way of making sense of your story and building an exciting vision for what's ahead.

A Joyful Purpose has three characteristics: it's authentic, important, and motivational. *Authentic* means the purpose has intrinsic buy-in from you. It's not what your culture or external influences tell you your purpose should be. *Important* means there's something at stake in the world if you don't live out this purpose. *Motivational* means the purpose gives you and other people joy.

You can define the Joyful Purpose behind your positive-change aspiration by answering these questions:

- **The Authentic Question:** Why is this aspiration part of your story?
- **The Important Question:** Why does this aspiration matter for the world and the people around you?
- **The Motivational Question:** Why does this aspiration excite you?

Following the example below, find the Joyful Purpose behind your positive-change aspirations.

ASPIRATION

Be debt free

WHY IS THIS ASPIRATION PART OF YOUR STORY?

My family struggled with debt growing up, and it stopped us from being financially generous.

WHY DOES THIS ASPIRATION MATTER FOR THE WORLD AND THE PEOPLE AROUND YOU?

If we become financially free, we can contribute more to the church and nonprofit ministries we care about.

WHY DOES THIS ASPIRATION EXCITE YOU?

I want to break the pattern of financial ignorance in my family. My children will know how to be good stewards who are generous with their money. They won't be held in financial bondage because of the choices I make.

JOYFUL PURPOSE

I want to become debt free so I can model to my kids what it looks like to be a good financial steward who makes the world better.

✔ Authentic
✔ Important
✔ Motivational

ASPIRATION

WHY IS THIS ASPIRATION PART OF YOUR STORY?

WHY DOES THIS ASPIRATION MATTER FOR THE WORLD AND THE PEOPLE AROUND YOU?

WHY DOES THIS ASPIRATION EXCITE YOU?

JOYFUL PURPOSE

☐ Authentic
☐ Important
☐ Motivational

ASPIRATION

WHY IS THIS ASPIRATION PART OF YOUR STORY?

**WHY DOES THIS ASPIRATION MATTER FOR THE WORLD
AND THE PEOPLE AROUND YOU?**

WHY DOES THIS ASPIRATION EXCITE YOU?

JOYFUL PURPOSE

☐ Authentic
☐ Important
☐ Motivational

ASPIRATION

WHY IS THIS ASPIRATION PART OF YOUR STORY?

**WHY DOES THIS ASPIRATION MATTER FOR THE WORLD
AND THE PEOPLE AROUND YOU?**

WHY DOES THIS ASPIRATION EXCITE YOU?

JOYFUL PURPOSE

☐ Authentic
☐ Important
☐ Motivational

ASPIRATION

WHY IS THIS ASPIRATION PART OF YOUR STORY?

WHY DOES THIS ASPIRATION MATTER FOR THE WORLD AND THE PEOPLE AROUND YOU?

WHY DOES THIS ASPIRATION EXCITE YOU?

JOYFUL PURPOSE

☐ Authentic
☐ Important
☐ Motivational

ASPIRATION

WHY IS THIS ASPIRATION PART OF YOUR STORY?

**WHY DOES THIS ASPIRATION MATTER FOR THE WORLD
AND THE PEOPLE AROUND YOU?**

WHY DOES THIS ASPIRATION EXCITE YOU?

JOYFUL PURPOSE

☐ Authentic
☐ Important
☐ Motivational

The purposes of

a person's heart

are deep waters,

but one who has insight

draws them out.

Proverbs 20:5

MAKE IT FUN

A deeper look at chapter 8 of Start from Joy

ONE OF MY (NEAL'S) FAVORITE JOBS WHEN I WAS IN COLLEGE was setting up and hosting construction-ministry youth camps across the country. One night I was in the back by the soundboard, and it was almost time to let the kids come rushing into the venue for a worship rally. I plugged in my iPod and turned on some Christian dance music. When the doors opened, the kids poured in, their excitement through the roof.

My team and I were excited too. While I stayed in the back to cue the music, my team members ran through the sanctuary pumping up the kids. I was dancing—if that's what you'd call my glorified sidestep (I'm known to bust a move, but I was keeping it tame).

That's when I saw an older adult approach me. I stopped my sidestep.

"We are in the house of the Lord," he said sternly. "Contain yourself."

He didn't let his eyes off me for the rest of the worship rally. My team members wondered why I wasn't pumping up the kids, but I was worried that if I moved one muscle wrong, this guy would find a way to get me fired. He seemed to hate the idea of me having fun at such a "serious" event.

Pleasure often gets a bad reputation, especially in Christian circles. We're told to deny fun in pursuit of a higher calling. But we forget that God is the one who created pleasure and fun in the first place. Psalm 37:4 tells us we were created to enjoy God. And Zephaniah 3:17 tells us that God enjoys us. To deny ourselves fun is to withhold God's good gifts in our life.

> God is the one who created pleasure and fun in the first place.

With our clients at Enjoyco, we often find that the struggle to have fun isn't just about beliefs. Trauma and pain, along with what we've been taught about fun, contribute to this struggle. When shame, guilt, and fear are present in our stories, it's difficult to feel safe enough to play and have fun.

Author Greg McKeown defines play as "anything we do simply for the joy of doing [it] rather than as a means to an end."[1] When everything we do revolves around an end goal, we know shame, guilt, and fear are behind our motivation. We go to the gym solely to lose weight. We avoid spending only to work on our bottom line. We put in endless hours at work to move up the ladder. There's no play in these endeavors.

> Play is anything we do simply for the joy of doing it.

Play brings us back to the joy of doing something without an end goal—moving our bodies for the fun of it, feeling safe to spend money, working because we enjoy our job. In this freedom, our greatest changes can occur. Why? Because we keep doing things we enjoy. If we bring fun and play into our endeavors, we will stick to them for the long term.

In the following group discussion questions and exercise, you'll learn to reclaim fun and play so you can enjoy positive change.

GROUP DISCUSSION QUESTIONS

1. Think about your relationship with fun. Do you struggle to enjoy yourself? Where do you think this view of fun came from?

2. When you imagine Jesus, do you picture him having fun? Why or why not? What would a joyful, fun-loving Jesus look like?

3. Think of someone you know who really enjoys life and has a lot of fun. How do people respond to that person? What do you think drives their joy?

4. In chapter 8 of *Start from Joy*, we talk about the importance of looking for fun. We often prime ourselves for change to be negative and difficult. How do your expectations influence what you experience?

5. Think about the activities you label "hard" or "not fun." How could you reframe these activities so you see them as more enjoyable?

6. When something great happens, do you celebrate? If so, how?

7. Are you able to celebrate little things, not just big milestones? If not, what holds you back?

8. Who celebrates your good news with you and validates your feelings?

9. How can you as a group help one another celebrate and have more fun?

A "What I Love List" (W.I.L.L., for short) is a tool to help you make positive actions more fun. It's exactly what it sounds like: a list of people, places, activities, and foods you love. Whenever you want to make a wise action more enjoyable, you can choose an item from this list and pair it with your positive action or use it as a reward. For instance, if you want to go for a run but struggle to make it happen, you might pair running with talking to someone from your list. Or if you have an overwhelming project at work, you can pair the project with a fun meal you listed on your W.I.L.L.

To begin, grab a notebook or open a document on your computer. Then list what you enjoy in the following categories.

- **People:** Who do you enjoy spending time with? Who do you enjoy talking to in person, on the phone, or over video chat?
- **Places:** Where do you enjoy going? Rather than thinking about vacation destinations or places you go only on occasion, consider places in your immediate vicinity. This could include locations such as your kitchen table or your porch or your favorite chair.
- **Activities:** What activities do you enjoy? This could be anything from going for a run to reading at your favorite coffee shop.
- **Food:** What foods do you enjoy? You could break your list down into food groups. What are your favorite vegetables? Fruits? Proteins? What meals do you enjoy cooking? What are your favorite restaurants?

Following the example below, you can create your own W.I.L.L.

Category	What I Love ♥
People	my small group from church
Place	the reading chair in my living room
Activity	walking outside
Food	buffalo wings

SAMPLE

Category	What I Love ♥

Category   **What I Love ♥**

Category   **What I Love ♥**

Category   **What I Love ♥**

Category	What I Love ♥

**Joy is the
serious business
of Heaven.**

C. S. Lewis

JOY FOR TODAY

A deeper look at chapters 9–12 of Start from Joy

PHILOSOPHER BLAISE PASCAL ONCE SAID that humans have a habit of turning nothing into eternity and eternity into nothing.[1] We are called to live in light of eternity—to set our minds on the things of heaven—but we often get distracted. Like the Israelites who worshiped a golden calf of their own creation,[2] we, too, get impatient for the joy and happiness of eternity. In doing so, we attach ourselves to false scripts that promise us happiness after we buy into their solution.

These false scripts not only deprive us of joy but create emotional patterns that keep us stuck. The things that don't have lasting significance become everything, and eternity gets banished to the recesses of our minds.

In our world of advertisements, materialism, and self-improvement, false scripts are everywhere. These scripts leave us exhausted and burned out, and they lead us away from positive change. But there's good news: we don't have to wait for eternity to experience happiness and joy. Joy is a fruit of the Spirit, which means we can have joy this side of heaven.[3]

Joy is available to us today, without having to change anything.

- How would it affect your life if you didn't feel pressured to change?
- What would open up for you if you took a gentler, lighter approach to change?
- What would your life look like if you were able to break your old patterns?

With a start-from-joy approach, we can stop trying so hard to achieve the change and happiness we want. We can embrace a lighter spirit and build a more fulfilling life. Best of all, we can keep eternity in perspective.

Pursuits such as organizing our finances, deepening our relationships, and prioritizing our health are good things. But God didn't create those good desires to replace eternity. Rather, eternity gives us a proper perspective on the other good things in our lives.

> Joy is available to us today, without having to change anything.

We steward our finances out of joy that God has given us everything we need. We deepen our relationships out of joy that God has given us these people to love and care for. We prioritize our health out of joy that God has given us capable bodies to navigate the world. When we live with eternity in mind, the fruit is joy. This allows us to lean into our present moment with gratitude and delight.

WRAP-UP QUESTIONS

1. What has changed in your life since you began your start-from-joy journey?

2. As you think back on the Negativity Loops you identified, which one was most eye-opening? How has this awareness changed the way you approach positive-change goals?

3. What is most challenging for you as you move away from shame, guilt, and fear as motivators for change?

4. What's one step you can take today to move forward in your start-from-joy journey?

RESOURCE: CAST A JOY VISION

The seven principles of a start-from-joy approach are not meant to be a step-by-step program. Rather, they're intended to push back against the different ways shame, guilt, and fear influence our journey to change. You can find value and experience change by implementing just one or two of the principles in this guidebook.

But what if you're ready to incorporate multiple principles into your positive-change journey?

The best way to start tying all seven principles together is to envision a future where you start from joy.

In your journal, write an entry that casts a vision for the future. Think of the area of your life where you most need to experience change. Then flesh out the scene of what it would look like to start from joy in that area.

- What will it look like and feel like when you're living out your Joyful Purpose in your positive-change journey?
- Instead of constantly hearing the voice of the Judge, what life-giving truths will you believe?
- What wise actions will you take when you feel shame, guilt, and fear?
- What will you do to have more fun in your life?

In a world of self-improvement, it's easy to believe that joy only comes after the hard work of change. But isn't it amazing that we don't have to hustle for joy? Jesus tells us that his yoke is easy and his burden is light.[4] This rest for our souls is available to us now.

Here's to living with joy *today*.

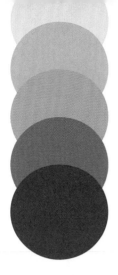

NOTES

SESSION 1: END THE MOTIVATION OF SHAME, GUILT, AND FEAR

1. Matthew 11:28-30, NLT.

SESSION 2: BE CURIOUS WITH YOUR EMOTIONS

1. Hebrews 2:17; 4:15.
2. John 11:1-44.
3. Matthew 21:12.
4. Matthew 26:38-39.
5. John 17:13.

SESSION 3: INTERRUPT YOUR LOOPS

1. Mark Grimsley, *Battle Films: Judgment at Nuremberg*, HistoryNet.com (March 6, 2018), https://www.historynet.com/battle-films-judgment-at-nuremberg.htm.
2. Andrew Glass, "600 Begin Selma-to-Montgomery March, March 7, 1965" (March 7, 2013), https://www.politico.com/story/2013/03/this-day-in-politics-088518.

3. Chris Simkins, *Non-violence Was Key to Civil Rights Movement*, VOANews.com (January 20, 2014), https://www.voanews.com/a/nonviolencekey-to-civil-rights -movement/1737280.html.

SESSION 4: CHALLENGE FALSE SCRIPTS

1. Matthew 6:33.

SESSION 5: CALL OUT THE JUDGE

1. Romans 8:1.
2. John 3:17.

SESSION 7: MAKE IT FUN

1. Greg McKeown, *Essentialism: The Disciplined Pursuit of Less* (New York: Currency, 2014), 85.

CONCLUSION: JOY FOR TODAY

1. Blaise Pascal, *Thoughts on Religion and Other Subjects* (Amherst, MA: J. S. and C. Adams, 1829), 76.
2. Exodus 32:1-6.
3. Galatians 5:22-23.
4. Matthew 11:28-30.

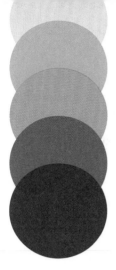

ABOUT THE AUTHORS

NEAL SAMUDRE is the cofounder and CEO of Enjoyco, an emotional health and wellness company designed to help individuals enjoy positive change. He is also a former marketing executive, where his leadership helped several Inc. 5000 companies scale. Neal is a viral writer on the subject of joy and positive psychology. More than five million people have shared his articles, and more than 500,000 people have completed his devotionals on the Bible App. Neal has been featured at the Catalyst Conference and in national publications such as *Relevant* magazine, *Church Leaders* magazine, *Huffington Post*, and more. He lives with his wife, Carly, and son, Jude, outside Nashville.

CARLY SAMUDRE, LPC-MHSP, is a licensed professional counselor in the greater Nashville area. She is also the cofounder of Enjoyco, an emotional health and wellness company that helps individuals enjoy positive change. In addition to her therapy practice, she is a sought-after speaker for women's ministries, leading women at all stages of their faith into deeper discipleship and biblical understanding. Carly holds a master's degree in clinical mental health counseling from Gordon-Conwell Theological Seminary. She lives outside Nashville with her husband, Neal, and their son, Jude.

SPACE FOR REFLECTION

SPACE FOR REFLECTION

SPACE FOR REFLECTION

SPACE FOR REFLECTION

SPACE FOR REFLECTION

SPACE FOR REFLECTION

Your successful, positive, and more joyful life starts now.

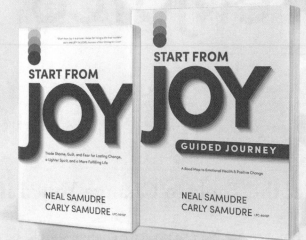

With *Start from Joy* and the *Start from Joy Guided Journey*, you'll:

- discover how you can use the gifts of joy to stick with positive change,
- develop a clearer picture of why your emotional patterns hold you back and how you can start making your emotions work for you, and
- heal your relationship with your body, work, money, and other people through easy, practical action steps.

Leave shame, guilt, and fear behind and create the fulfilling life you were always meant to live!

www.enjoyco.com

enjoyco

Get the Tools to Change Your Life

At Enjoyco, we believe positive change should be a clear and enjoyable experience. Through our tools and teachings, we simplify emotional health and wellness so you can create lasting change.

If you loved the tools we mentioned in the book, get access to them and more at . . .

enjoycowellness.com/sfj